DASHERS FOR ANTI-AGING

*Non-secret organic delicious yummy smoothies for
all seasons to make you look younger and healthier*

AVA COLLINS

Disclaimer

The content of this book is designed to give you a helpful
information on the ways to regain your beautiful skin and body using
raw fruits and vegetables into delicious and healthy beneficial
smoothies.

TABLE OF CONTENTS

SUMMARY

Researchers found that the process of aging is accelerated by some special particular molecules named free radicals. They collide with cells present in our body, sucking them of their electrons that accelerate aging. However, there are ways to control these molecules – "antioxidants". They offer some extra electrons to the free radicals that neutralizes them. Wonderful thing about antioxidants is that they are easy easily found in food. Most vegetables and fruits are likely to contain rich antioxidants. It's not that simple to eat the same fruit as a lot, but it's better easier to make use of them in the form of smoothies.

Even if you blame your mom or call it as a bad genetic issue—don't forget that you have to consider that your complexion is shown out only with what you are eating. As seen and said in ancient times, eating healthy foods in a right way has a direct impact on your appearance, like an old saying "you are what you eat," actually is a fact. So, instead of simply checking your skin for worrying in the wash towel, bring out your blender, and keep whipping up one of these smoothies on a regular basis that will result in sprucing your complexion in no-time.

I have always been on a smoothie not only in summer, but for my everyday routine it's my breakfast after a workout, besides a great way to clear out my fridge. Rather than having juices, smoothies help in utilizing the whole fruit and vegetables which retain all the nutrients in the skin and consumes more fiber to keep you full longer. To learn how to make simple miracle resulting anti-aging delicious smoothies just follow the below natural colorful dashers and see drastic change in your skin and body.

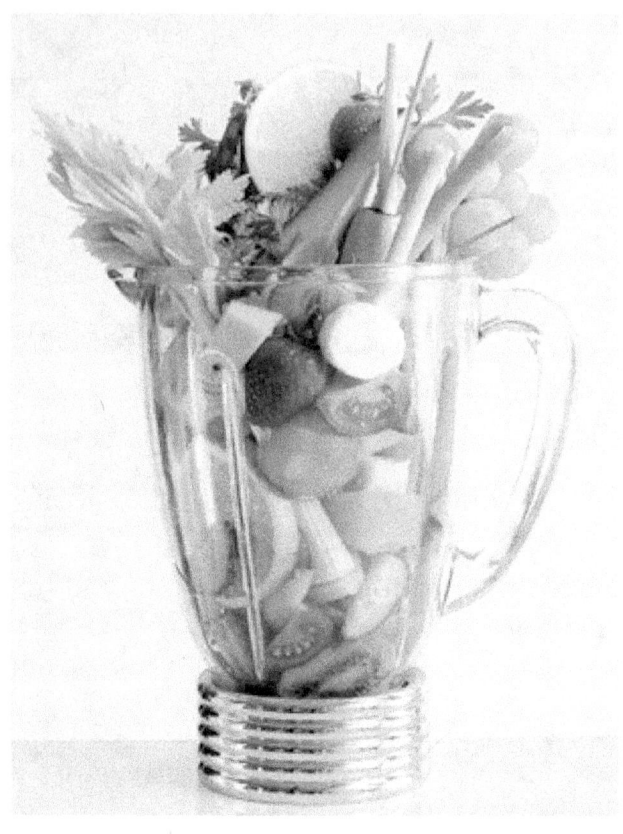

The beauty is not any facial mode but the true beauty is reflected in our soul. It is the 'caring' that we love to give the passion that we show. The beauty actually grows with the passing years if we bring out our passion that inspires us and also the

people around us. Beauty is nothing but a power that brings a smile as its sword.

We people are like stained glass windows that shine and sparkle in sun rays and when the sun sets out, the true beauty is revealed out only if there is a light within us. This book is inspired to bring that light of beauty hidden in us with some simple and easy possible ways.

Spinach and Pear Smoothie

This smoothie is inspired by a mouthwatering salad that I love. Though there is some spinach in it, you'd never be able to tell, because it's is sweet and tastes amazing. It's a great fix for those times when you are craving something sweet. With the fiber, iron, and vitamin C that this drink offers, you will never have to feel guilty about giving in.

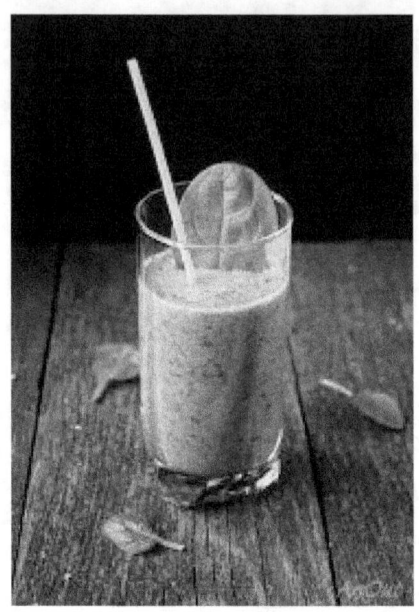

Ingredients:

6 small pears

1 tablespoon raisins

4 cups baby spinach

2 tablespoons fresh lemon juice

1 cup filtered water

2 cups ice

<u>Yield:</u> 2 servings

Combine all ingredients, except the ice, and nutmeg, in a blender, and puree until smooth. Taste and add sweetener if required. If a thicker and cooler smoothie is desired, blend in some crushed ice. Top with some dashers of your choice.

Cherry Smoothie

Fresh cherries are so amazing! If you are lucky enough to get your hands on some sweet dark cherries, you will be delighted to know that you are fortifying your body with a ton of antioxidants. Yummy and healthy!

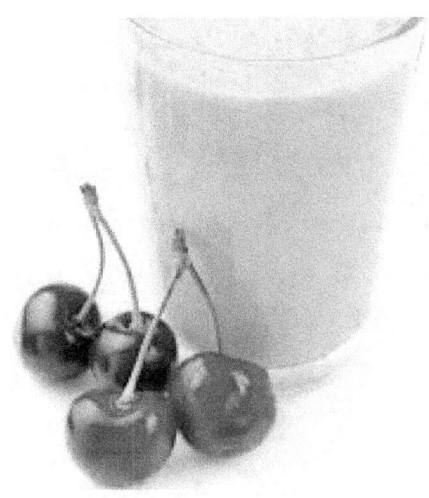

Ingredients:

3 cups pitted sweet cherries

2 tablespoons shredded unsweetened coconut

1 1/2 cups unsweetened almond milk

2/3 cup unsalted raw almonds

1 ½ medium bananas

1 cup ice

Yield: 2 servings

Combine all ingredients, except the ice, and nutmeg, in a blender, and puree until smooth. Taste and add sweetener if required. If a thicker and cooler smoothie is desired, blend in some crushed ice. Top with some dashers of your choice.

Green Tea, Grape, Apple and Spinach Smoothie

My girlfriends love this one. If you are a green tea lover, you will go crazy too. Amazing flavor of the spinach and tea perfectly as well as sweetness of grapes are wonderful. This smoothie also contains tons of minerals.

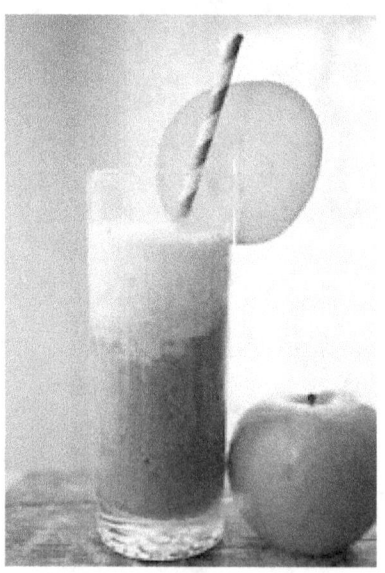

Ingredients:

1 1/2 cups cooled strong green tea

3 cups green grapes

1 green apple

2 cups baby spinach

2 cups ice

Yield: 2 servings

Combine all ingredients, except the ice, and nutmeg, in a blender, and puree until smooth. Taste and add sweetener if required. If a thicker and cooler smoothie is desired, blend in some crushed ice. Top with some dashers of your choice.

Carrot and Mango Smoothie

The flavor profile of a mango is complex. People can detect peach, orange or even carrot. And herein is the key to its lovely taste. By adding carrots you make it even more delicious.

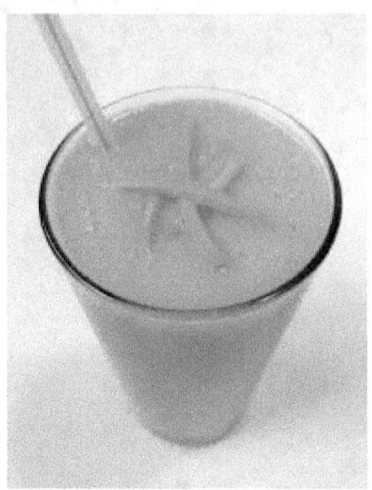

Ingredients:

2 medium mangoes, peeled and pitted

1 small carrot, peeled

2 tablespoons unsweetened shredded coconut

2 tablespoons freshly squeezed lime juice

1 cup filtered water

2 cups ice

Yield: 2 servings

Combine all ingredients, except the ice, and nutmeg, in a blender, and puree until smooth. Taste and add sweetener if required. If a thicker and cooler smoothie is desired, blend in some crushed ice. Top with some dashers of your choice.

Grape Smoothie

Even though there are few ingredients, this smoothie is delicious. Thanks to rosemary if tastes even better.

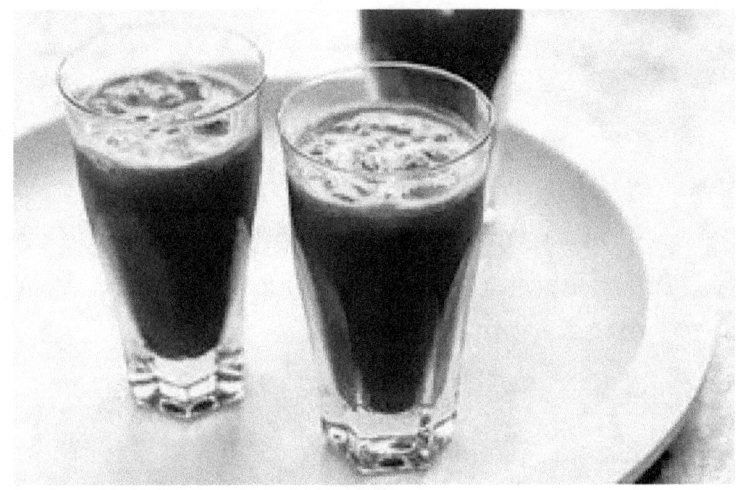

Ingredients:

4 cups red grapes

1 teaspoon fresh rosemary leaves

2 red apples

1 cup ice

Yield: 2 servings

Combine all ingredients, except the ice, and nutmeg, in a blender, and puree until smooth. Taste and add sweetener if required. If a thicker and cooler smoothie is desired, blend in some crushed ice. Top with some dashers of your choice.

Mango Smoothie

There are not many exotic smoothies out there and, frankly, sometimes they are horrible. I might be wrong but this smoothie is definitely delicious.

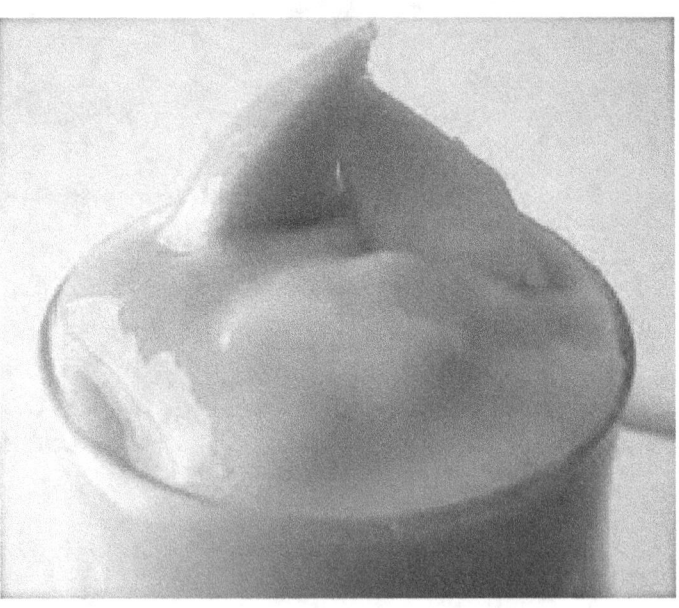

Ingredients:

2 medium mangoes, peeled and pitted

1/2 teaspoon ground turmeric

2 teaspoons juice of lime

8 dates

2 cups unsweetened almond milk

2 cups ice

Yield: 2 servings

Combine all ingredients, except the ice, and nutmeg, in a blender, and puree until smooth. Taste and add sweetener if required. If a thicker and cooler smoothie is desired, blend in some crushed ice. Top with some dashers of your choice.

Cocoa Banana

Polyphones from cacao are antioxidants that protect the body from oxidizing agents and can protect the skin and cells.

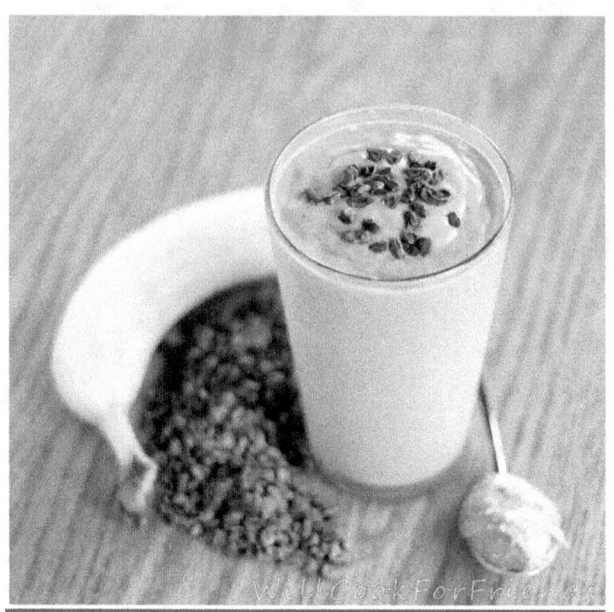

Ingredients:

2 banana

10 strawberries

1 Tablespoon cacao powder (polyphones)

1 cup unsweetened milk

Yield: 2 servings

Combine all ingredients, except the ice, and nutmeg, in a blender, and puree until smooth. Taste and add sweetener if required. If a thicker and cooler smoothie is desired, blend in some crushed ice. Top with some dashers of your choice.

Tropical Smoothie

As we age, our skin loses its moisture and elasticity which causes more wrinkles. Omega-3s have been found to provide the skin with more moisture by keeping the cells of the epidermis (our top layer of skin) plump and hydrated.

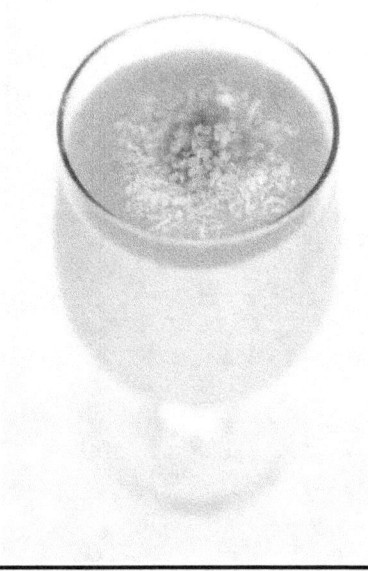

Ingredients:
1 cup mango (sliced)
2 cup pineapple (sliced)
1 Tablespoon Chia seeds (Omega-3)
1 cup coconut water

Yield: 2 servings

Combine all ingredients, except the ice, and nutmeg, in a blender, and puree until smooth. Taste and add sweetener if required. If a thicker and cooler smoothie is desired, blend in some crushed ice. Top with some dashers of your choice.

Vitamin-E Green Smoothie

Vitamin E helps the skin retain moisture and protects it from the harmful effects of free radicals.

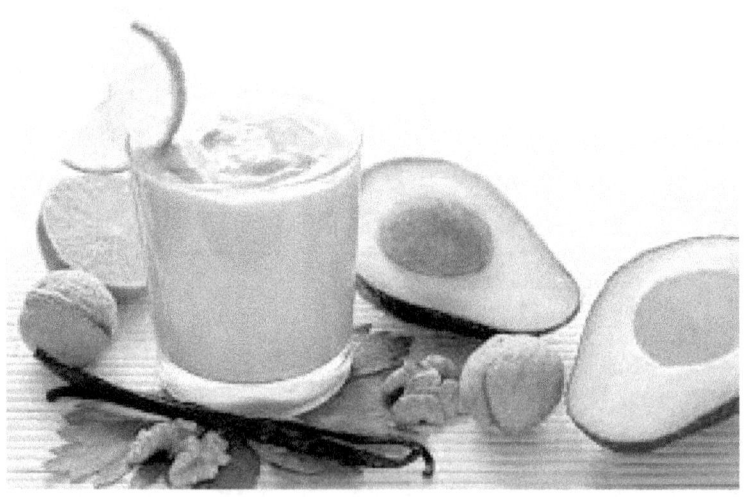

Ingredients:
2 cup of tightly packed spinach (vitamin E)

1 ripe medium banana
4 Tablespoons avocado (peeled and pit removed) (vitamin E)
1 Tablespoon sunflower seeds (vitamin E)
4 Tablespoons lemon juice
1 cup of unsweetened almond milk (vitamin E)

Yield: 2 servings

Combine all ingredients, except the ice, and nutmeg, in a blender, and puree until smooth. Taste and add sweetener if required. If a thicker and cooler smoothie is desired, blend in some crushed ice. Top with some dashers of your choice.

Breeze of Blueberry

I am not sure how I've come up with this recipe, but I can definitely say that it is one of the best I've ever tried. Vitamin C improves cell growth and one study even suggested a diet high in vitamin C can result in fewer wrinkles. Vitamin C also helps regenerate other vitamins in the body like Vitamin E.

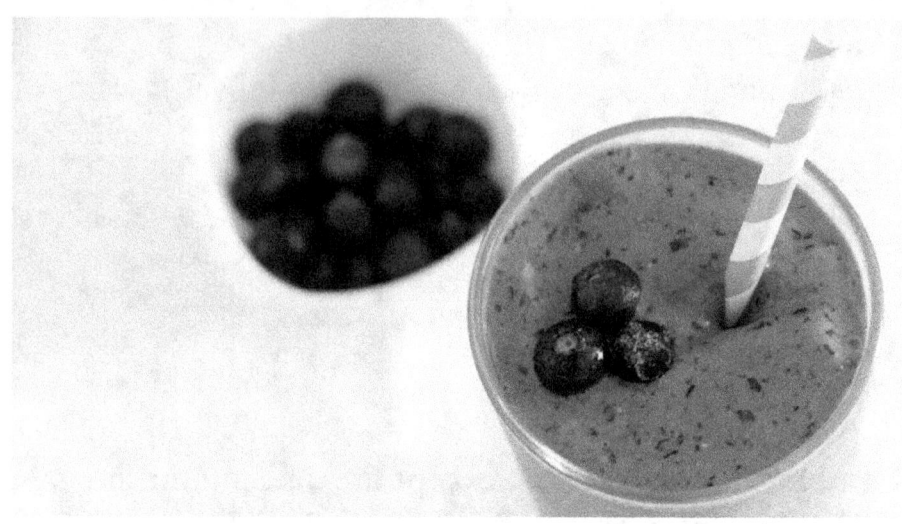

Ingredients:
2 cup fresh or frozen blueberries (vitamin C)
2 cup fresh or frozen strawberries (vitamin C)
1 cup coconut water
2 Tablespoon lemon juice (vitamin C)
1 teaspoon chia seeds
1 handful of mint (leaves only) (vitamin C)

<u>Yield:</u> 2 servings

Combine all ingredients, except the ice, and nutmeg, in a blender, and puree until smooth. Taste and add sweetener if required. If a thicker and cooler smoothie is desired, blend in some crushed ice. Top with some dashers of your choice.

Kale and Carrot Smoothie

Beta-Carotene, a carotenoid antioxidant, protects cells from damage and assists with better eyesight, too.

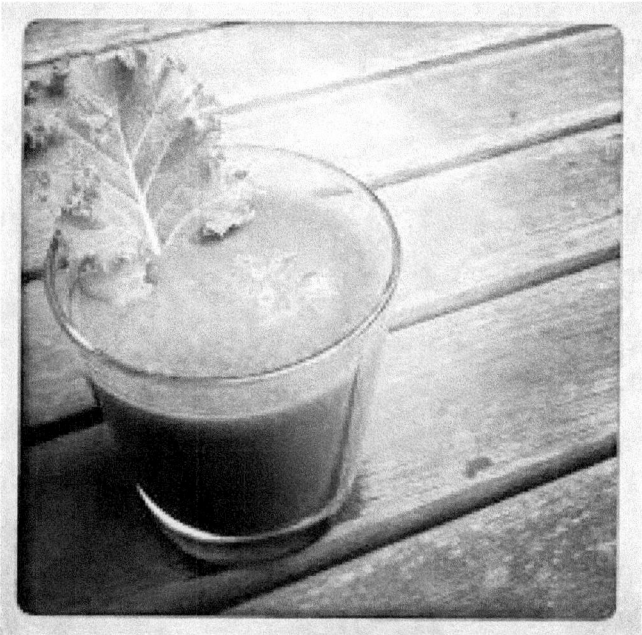

Ingredients:
2 cup kale (only take the leaf part and leave out the stem) (beta-carotene)
2 carrot (chopped) (beta-carotene)
1 green apple (core removed and chopped)
Lemon juice from 1 lemon or 2 Tablespoons lemon juice
1 cup coconut water

Yield: 2 servings

Combine all ingredients, except the ice, and nutmeg, in a blender, and puree until smooth. Taste and add sweetener if required. If a thicker and cooler smoothie is desired, blend in some crushed ice. Top with some dashers of your choice.

Clear Skin Smoothie

Not only do the ingredients in the clean, green smoothie revitalize your skin with antioxidants that promote cell renewal thanks to the spinach, cucumber, celery, and parsley, they also provide a quick detox and energy boost. Pre-make this one and bring along to work for an afternoon pick-me-up.

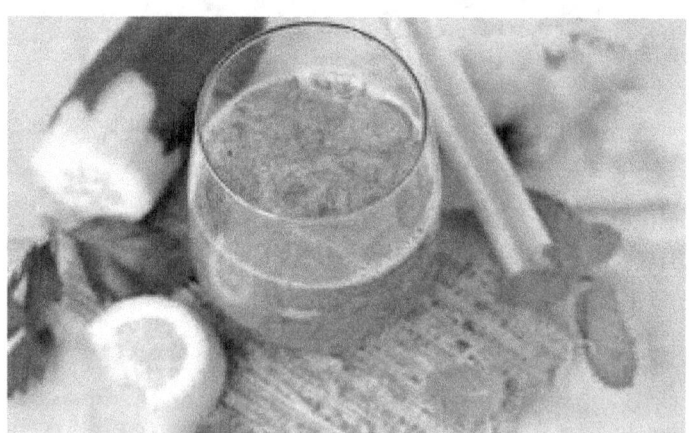

INGREDIENTS:

1 an avocado

2 cup of fresh spinach

1 teaspoon of coconut oil (up it to a tablespoon if you prefer!)

1 small bunch of parsley

1 cucumber, sliced

1 or 2 stalks of celery

juice from 1/2 a lime, squeezed

1 cup of room temperature water

Yield: 2 servings

Combine all ingredients, except the ice, and nutmeg, in a blender, and puree until smooth. Taste and add sweetener if required. If a thicker and cooler smoothie is desired, blend in some crushed ice. Top with some dashers of your choice.

Coconut Water Smoothie

Looking to try some of the most sought-after ingredients found in the best skin products but in a smoothie? Then look no further! The following recipe whips up this coconut water-based smoothie that will rehydrate your skin. Added bonuses include strawberries to assist in collagen production, carrots providing anti-aging oxidants and the oranges encouraging cell rejuvenation.

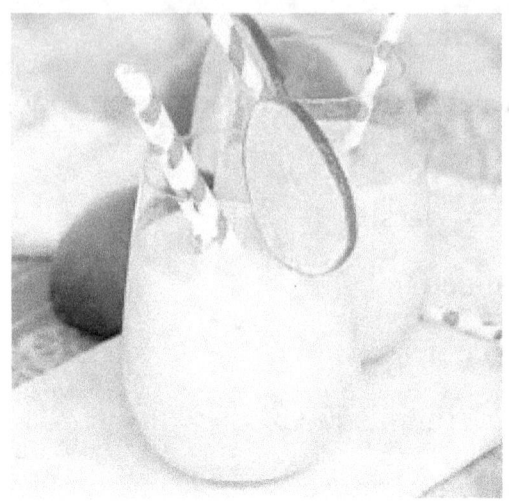

Ingredients:

2 cup coconut water, chilled

2 cup fresh or frozen organic strawberries

2 cup organic baby carrots

2 cup fresh or frozen mango chunks

1 navel orange, peeled

<u>Yield:</u> 2 servings

Combine all ingredients, except the ice, and nutmeg, in a blender, and puree until smooth. Taste and add sweetener if required. If a thicker and cooler smoothie is desired, blend in some crushed ice. Top with some dashers of your choice.

Banana Almond Flax Smoothie

Flax seeds are fabulous for your skin—fighting against irritation, redness, and inflammation— while the vitamin E found in almonds help rid your body of toxins and the vitamins A, B, and E in bananas are excellent anti-aging properties. This Cookie and Kate smoothie combines the power of all of these ingredients for one skin smoothing smoothie.

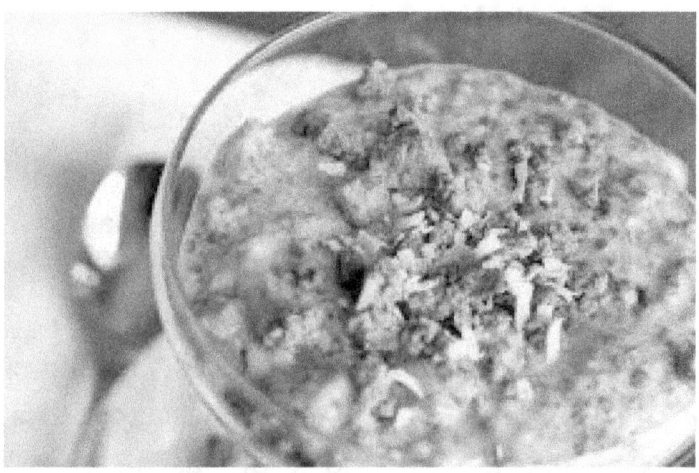

Ingredients:

2 medium or large frozen bananas, broken into one-inch chunks before frozen

2 heaping spoonful of almond butter

2 spoonfuls of flax seed

1 cup of almond milk (can alternate with yogurt or whole milk)

a drizzle of honey (or agave nectar or maple syrup)

a small drop of almond extract (or vanilla extract)

Yield: 2 servings

Combine all ingredients, except the ice, and nutmeg, in a blender, and puree until smooth. Taste and add sweetener if required. If a thicker and cooler smoothie is desired, blend in some crushed ice. Top with some dashers of your choice.

Bee Pollen Smoothie

Blueberries and bee pollen are the ultimate anti-wrinkle combo—you'll be looking as wrinkle-free as you have in *forever* with this recipes from Healthy Bee pollen is an anti-aging super food that battles free radicals and prevents signs of premature aging like wrinkles and under-eye circles. It also supports the cardiovascular system, improves digestion and strengthens the immune system. So drink up!

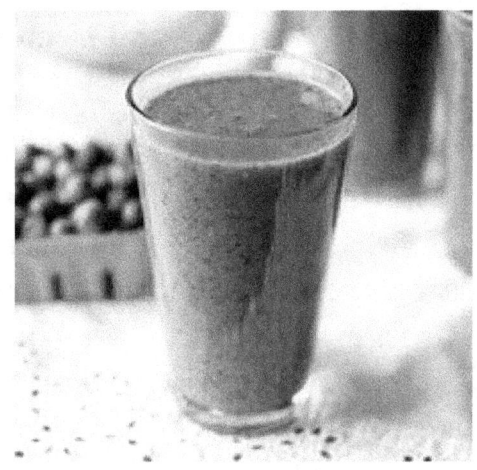

Ingredients:

2 cup of almond or coconut milk

2 cup of frozen blueberries

1 fresh or frozen medium-sized banana

1 tablespoon of bee pollen

1 tablespoon of coconut oil

A dollop of honey or maple syrup, optional

Yield: 2 servings

Combine all ingredients, except the ice, and nutmeg, in a blender, and puree until smooth. Taste and add sweetener if required. If a thicker and cooler smoothie is desired, blend in some crushed ice. Top with some dashers of your choice.

Parsley, Cucumber, Pineapple and Lemon Smoothie

This super healthy smoothie is surprisingly sweet and so yummy, made with absolutely no dairy – delicious! "Parsley is brilliant for alleviating inflammation, asthma and airborne allergies. This blend's mineral salts neutralizes acids, purifies blood, cleanses skin, detoxifies tissues and organs, assists with elimination of heavy metals, flushes out kidneys and aids in urinary tract health."

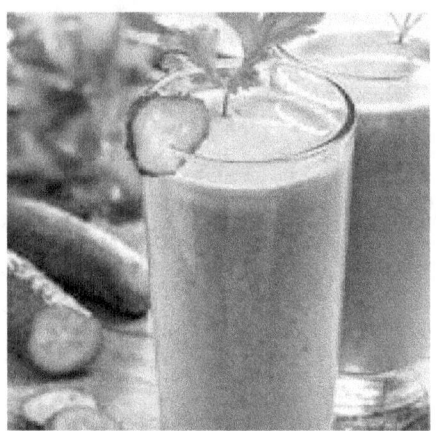

Ingredients:

1 cup coconut water (or water)

1 big size cucumber, chopped

2 bunches of flat leaf parsley, leaves only, chopped

2 medium lemons, peeled and seeded

2 cups frozen pineapple

5 drops liquid stevia, or more to taste

Combine all ingredients, except the ice, and nutmeg, in a blender, and puree until smooth. Taste and add sweetener if required. If a thicker and cooler smoothie is desired, blend in some crushed ice. Top with some dashers of your choice.

Kiwi Smoothie

Kiwis are a rich source of vitamin C. They are also a good source of vitamins A (as beta-carotene), B6, E and K as well as foliate, magnesium, phosphorus, copper and dietary fiber. The edible seeds contain omega-3 fatty acids. Antioxidants are especially present in the skin, which you can leave on the fruit as long as it is organic. Kiwifruit contains actinide, which is an enzyme that breaks down protein.

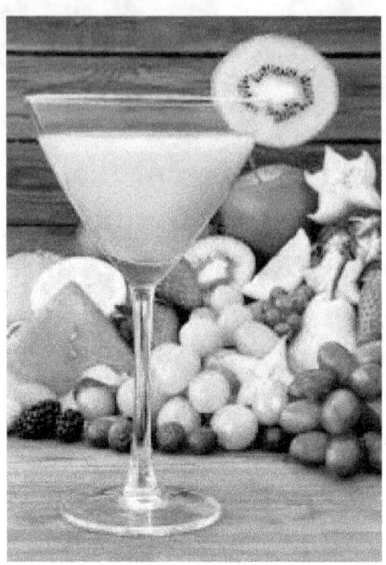

Ingredients:

4 kiwis
1 banana or apple or 1 cup strawberries
2 cups fresh baby spinach (or other leafy green)
1/2 avocado
1 cup water

Yield: 2 servings

Combine all ingredients, except the ice, and nutmeg, in a blender, and puree until smooth. Taste and add sweetener if required. If a thicker and cooler smoothie is desired, blend in some crushed ice. Top with some dashers of your choice.

Many Varieties of super foods gifted by our nature contains powerful nutrients that will actually help in keeping signs of aging at bay. Particular, many raw fruits and vegetables lend a juicy concentration of valuable vitamins, beauty minerals, and dietary antioxidants, leading to the "the real natural beauty intakes" of this edible world. Super food smoothies are a key way to consume this beneficial spectrum of anti-aging powerhouses. For best results, aim for smoothies that are high in antioxidant foods, rich in fresh produce, include healthy fats, and use plenty of purified water.

Bring your real beauty out by having these nature give beauty products. Stay young and healthy by regaining your gorgeous skin and body that makes you love yourself and inspire others.

If you loved this book and found it useful I would be very glad if you post a short review. I read all the reviews personally so I can get your feedback and make this book even better.

THANK YOU

AVA COLLINS

www.ingramcontent.com/pod-product-compliance
Lightning Source LLC
Chambersburg PA
CBHW060349290526
45791CB00004B/1601